Your Ar
Itty B.
Heal Your Body Book

15 Essential Steps to Heal our Mind, Body and Spirit

Are you overwhelmed or tired? Do you feel overweight or lack a sense of well-being? Can you find time to exercise and meet your own needs? Are you living your purpose and dream?

If you desire more vibrant life force energy, a healthier mind and body and a more joyful life lived with purpose, start now and follow the tips in this Itty Bitty book.

- "Thanks to Patricia I was able to integrate fitness into my lifestyle as an older adult" - Andrea Adelson.
- "Thank you so much for bringing us to a higher level of fitness and awareness, we are forever grateful." Jami and Dennis Hensling
- "Patricia Garza changed my life when I needed it the most. She was there for me as much more than a great trainer." Jackie Cunningham

If you want to begin your healing journey pick up a copy of this simple ground breaking book today!

Your Amazing
Itty Bitty®
Heal Your Body Book

15 Simple Steps to Healing Your Body, Mind and Spirit

Patricia Garza Pinto

Published by Itty Bitty® Publishing
A subsidiary of S & P Productions, Inc.

Printed in the United States of America

Itty Bitty® Publishing
311 Main Street, Suite D
El Segundo, CA 90245
(310) 640-8885

ISBN: 978-1-931191-57-9

Dedication

I dedicate this book to several people near and dear t my heart:

Wayne Daniels, my dear friend. Wayne, thank you for guiding me through my holistic healing process and spiritual evolution.

Paul Check of the world renown CHEK Institute and author of **How To Eat, Move and Be Healthy.** Paul, thank you for living your purpose and dream and for sharing your love and wisdom with the world. Without you following your dream, part of me feels I would have never have discovered mine. Love and chi to you, my beloved teacher!

Merijildo Garza - Dad, thanks for being my initial teach in the file of fitness and exercise. I appreciate my experience of you dragging me into the hot, sticky, sweaty, testosterone-infused "men's side of the gym" to become a student of exercise and fitness approximately 42 years ago.

www.DIVINEMOUNTAINRETREAT.com

Stop by our Itty Bitty® website to find interesting information about healing your body at:

www.IttyBittyPublishing.com

Or visit Patricia Garza Pinto at:

www.DIVINEMOUNTAINRETREAT.com

patriciawholistic@gmail.com

For a FREE consultation call:
+1-949-422-1168

Table of Contents

Disclaimer: This Itty Bitty™ Heal Your Body booklet is written and designed to assist in healing your body, mind and spirit and not meant to diagnose or cure illness.

Introduction

In this Itty Bitty™ Book you will discover 15 easy steps to follow daily which will assist in opening up your body's energy healing channels. Our bodies were designed to heal themselves, despite what your doctor tells you! Therefore, you have a choice to experience life to your fullest potential or end up dis-eased, broken and decrepit.

In my experience, if we are not resting, eating well, exercising or know our purpose and dream, we are merely existing and not living up to our purest potential.

From this moment forward I ask you to commit to choose a life of vibrant health and well-being.

Simple Steps

Step 1
Rest Is Imperative

Are you taking time to be still and rest or does your life involve hectic, chaotic days?

1. Proper rest is an important role in assisting to heal the body. After all, how can we feel good enough to live our purpose and dream without sufficient rest and recovery?
2. If you do not take the time to rest your body, your body will constantly be in the fight or flight mode, which is likened to being chased by a vicious tiger – there is no peace and rest in the fight or flight mode.
3. Honor yourself and rest up, my friend!

Tips For More Restful Days

- Get organized: clean out the clutter in your *life*, This means your physical, mental and spiritual closet.
- Allow yourself guilt-free time to sit or lie down for some much needed quiet time – at least 10-20 minutes per day.
- If you have a baby or small children, perhaps you would consider resting or sitting silently while they are napping or watching their favorite educational program on TV.
- Listen to peaceful, mellow music to soothe your soul.
- Take time to rest with a warm cup of chamomile or other soothing, non-caffeinated tea.
- Consider a slow, easy walk outside in nature.
- Take a break from unnecessary noise or distractions, i.e., television and radio.
- Commit to at least 5 minutes of stillness and quiet with several "quiet/rest" sessions throughout the day.
- Give yourself *permission* to rest!

Step 2
Sleep For Better Performance

For our mind, body and spirit to function properly, our bodies require adequate sleep. Lack of proper sleep means we may experience brain fog, lack of clarity, less focus, and age sooner. Poor sleep patterns mean more health problems. Proper sleep is imperative to optimally experience the other steps included in this Itty Bitty™ Book.

1. Do you feel you sleep soundly and properly? Disrupted sleep cycles affect hormonal levels.
    a. You should sleep between the hours of 10pm and 6am.
    b. Sleep between the hours of 10pm and 2am repairs your physical body.
    c. Between 2am and 6am, your body promotes psychological repair.
2. Adequate sleep means better regulated hormonal patterns in your body and with better sleep, comes increased feelings of well-being.

I trust you now understand the importance of a good night's sleep!

Tips For Better Sleep

- One hour before bedtime, dim ALL bright lights – consider using candles.
- Turn off noisy/busy distractions by 9:30pm. T.V., radio, people and, if necessary, quiet any barking dogs.
- After lunch and before bedtime, cut out ALL stimulants such as coffee, caffeinated teas and drinks, alcoholic beverages, sugar-filled junk foods and unhealthy snacks.
- Perform gentle stretching before bed. This means arms stretched overhead and legs at shoulder width and fully stretched and hold for 30 seconds. Repeat six to ten times with deep belly breaths.
- Have a hot bath or shower. Just not too hot!
- Try to block out any light in your bedroom.
- Try not to sleep in after 6am or you may get too much sleep, which will continue to disrupt your natural sleep rhythms.
- Stick to a sleep schedule: In bed for sleep by 10pm, sleeping through 6am.
- Move away from or turn off any EMF's (electro-magnetic fields): television, radio, smart phones, i-Pads, i-Pods, laptops and other devices.

Step 3
Meditate Your Way To Peace And Well-being

Meditation has been around for thousands of years and is widely used by many different cultures.

1. One need not sit in a pretzel-style lotus position to meditate. You may meditate while:
    a. lying in bed, on a comfy sofa or in your favorite chaise lounge chair.
    b. All that is required is an open mind and a quiet meditation spot.
2. Some of the many benefits of meditation are: boosts immune function; decreases pain, anxiety and depression; increases positive feel-good emotions; improves sleep; increases awareness; regulates blood pressure; improves feel-good moods and decreases tension.
3. Meditation is prescribed to Marines and other soldiers to facilitate a sense of peace and well-being. I trust it will be good enough to calm *your* spirit!

Tips For Meditation

- Choose something to focus or meditate on (serene location or gentle, soothing music).
- Schedule time to meditate regularly – a consistent time each day.
- Pick a quiet meditation spot at home or a quiet location out in nature.
- If you choose a quiet room at home, turn out the lights and light a candle - or just dim the lights.
- Choose to meditate in pure silence or listen to some peaceful, soothing music – no lyrics, just gentle music/melody.
- Make yourself comfortable – lie on the bed, sofa, or floor, or sit up with straight posture in a comfy chair. If you are lying down supine, you may fall asleep, and that's ok!
- If you sit in a chair, gently place your hands on your knees or in your lap.
- Close your eyes and take some deep belly breaths before your meditation session.
- If you have "monkey mind" and find it difficult to get out of your busy thoughts, focus on your belly breaths – this will keep you focused on breath, not your busy brain.
- Start small, beginning with 3-5 minutes per day, and work your way up to longer periods of meditation time.
- Get into a mental zone – learn to clear the mind of busy distractions. You can do this by focusing and repeating this affirmation; *I am happy, I am healthy, I am whole*

Step 4
Prayer Time For Divine Connection

Allow me to keep this section simple: prayer is an authentic request for help or offering thanks to God, Divine Source, Great Spirit or the Universe – a heavenly, divine connection to something greater than ourselves.

1. The effects of prayer are proven to offset negative health effects of stress and regulate your heartbeat for healthier heart function.
2. Prayer promotes relaxation and improves health and well-being. As you put your ego aside, let go and surrender to something greater than yourself, open up to the power of the mighty Universe for healing, health and well-being.
3. There is more to the world we live in than meets the eye. Prayer connects us to a universal Divine Source/God.
4. In my experience, prayer is also known to promote positive well-being, keeping you emotionally and spiritually grounded.

Prayer Tips

- For your prayer time, find a quiet, peaceful spot where you will not be interrupted.
- Set your intention: what do you want from this prayer session? Ask for it from your heart.
- Have an open mind and heart – be open and accepting.
- Set a time limit of at least five minutes a day – time to be with God/Divine Source/Great Spirit/Goddess.
- Engage a prayer partner and pray together ("where two or more are gathered," strong intentions are set and magic happens).
- Pray for others as it takes the focus off your own negativity.
- Offer thanks and gratitude for your life, every breath and heartbeat.
- Pray out loud – make your voice heard while opening your heart to your deepest intention.
- Sing your prayers – make your prayer into a song.
- Join a prayer group.

Step 5
Foods - Vibrant Life Force Wholesome Energy

I trust most of society (based on major health issues many Americans suffer) has little or no understanding and appreciation of the importance of healthy, wholesome foods. How can we heal our body, mind and spirit if we fill ourselves with less than optimal food?

1. My personal rule is: eat as close to "real" food as possible.
2. What is "real" food? Real food is non-processed, chemical laden "fake" foods or "Frankenfoods."
3. Real foods are grown on a local farm. They include: vegetables, fruits and farm-raised animals.
4. Pure, wholesome foods have natural, vibrant life force energy and as we eat more of them, we also begin to obtain more powerful life force energy from these same foods.
5. If we stuff our gullets with dead, highly processed foods, we should expect to feel less than optimal. This means ditching the junk food and foods with toxic chemical additives as they are ultimately dangerous and unhealthy for our body and mind.

Tips For More Optimal Food Choices

- Use healthy cooking oils: Ghee (clarified butter), olive oil, coconut oil, red palm oil.
- Always buy organic – eat more fruits and veggies.
- Avoid GMO (genetically modified organism) or "Frankenfoods" (buy non-GMO foods).
- Avoid the inner isles at your local supermarkets as the shelves are filled with fake, highly processed and chemically-filled foods.
- Consider eating a variety of healthy foods you do not normally eat – step outside the box.
- Start your day by eating a healthy, wholesome, organic balanced breakfast.
- Buy high quality protein: grass-fed, pasture-raised, wild-caught.
- Ditch sugary drinks like soda, shakes and high sugar energy drinks.
- Avoid ALL gluten products/foods.
- Do not buy pasteurized foods and drinks (these are "dead" foods).
- Buy local produce grown in your own state.
- Avoid: Mazola, corn, Canola and vegetable oils, as well as fake butters and margarine.
- Be aware of all organic processed foods as they are NOT optimal and lack vitality.

Step 6
Organic vs. Conventional Foods

I would suggest you avoid conventional foods at all cost and spend your hard-earned money on organic foods!

1. What are conventional foods? Conventional foods are foods and animals which are grown and raised by farming methods employing herbicides, pesticides, fungicides, antibiotics and hormones.

2. What are organic foods? Organic foods are grown by organic farming methods, naturally - without toxic chemicals and pesticides - in clean organic soil. Synthetic pesticides and chemical fertilizers are not allowed in organic foods.

3. There is no way ingesting herbicides, pesticides, fungicides, antibiotics and hormones can be healthy! Would you consciously choose to pump your body with these toxins? If not, why buy them in the supermarket and eat them?

Tips For Buying Organic Foods

- Buy organic seedlings and consider growing some of your own produce.
- Set the intention for your shopping trip to only purchase organic items.
- Learn to read labels and refrain from purchasing food items with ingredients you cannot understand or pronounce.
- Buy organic items which are stamped with a "certified organic" seal of approval.
- Find local farmers markets to shop.
- Ask your local supermarket manager if they sell organic items.
- If your supermarket does not sell organic, find one that does or request the store manager to start stocking organic items.
- Eat organic produce soon after purchasing as it will rot quickly (due to lack of chemicals and dangerous sprays. Organic produce does not last long).
- Buy in season when produce is most optimal in nutrition and flavor.
- Join a food co-op, as their produce is more affordable and seasonal.

Step 7
Conventional Foods

In conventional farming, animals are forced to live in unnatural and inhumane, cramped conditions. Conventionally-farmed animals are also given antibiotics and hormones. As you understand the conditions these animals are kept in, you may decide to support your local organic farms and farmers.

1. Animals living in conventional conditions suffer greatly as these animals are, by nature, meant to graze on natural grasses out in the sunlight. They are also fed unnatural toxic blends of hormones, chemicals, unhealthy fillers (such as wood pulp), GMO grains and soy, along with blood and body parts from other animals.

2. Due to the inhumane living conditions, many of the animals get sick; therefore, all are treated with antibiotics to avoid illness.

3. Remember: everything the animals ingest, you ingest!

Tips For Buying Sustainable Foods

- Support your local farmer(s).
- Discover where your local farmers sell their products - buy local foods and produce.
- Shop at farmer's markets over the mega-chain grocery superstores.
- Ask your local supermarket manager if they sell sustainable foods. If so, BUY THEM!
- Consider growing your own produce.
- Buy foods in bulk. You can get legumes, nuts, herbs, etc., for easy storing.
- Choose wild-caught seafood over farm-raised.
- Consider fermenting and canning or jarring your own foods.
- Buy animal proteins from your local farmer or from purveyors at your local farmers market.

Step 8
Water - The Importance of Hydrating

Our bodies are made up of approximately 50-80% water, depending on the amount of fat your body contains.

1. That stated, it is imperative we hydrate properly to assist in the body's daily functions.
2. You should consume half your body weight in ounces of pure, high quality water daily.
3. The health benefits of water include: better mental clarity, more vibrant - healthier looking skin, less puffiness and bloating; less constipation; better sleep; more energy and better physical performance.
4. Ice water can interfere with the body's ability to digest food properly. I suggest you drink room temperature or cool water on hot, warm days while exercising.

Tips For Water Consumption

- Drink 8 ounces of pure water upon awakening.
- Make a commitment to yourself to increase your daily water intake.
- If you have the financial means, purchase a good quality water filtration system for your home.
- Buy a small water filtration system (e.g., Brita). It is affordable and better than over-the-counter fluoridated tap water.
- Purchase a 24oz. size water bottle or half gallon of water to take with you at all times.
- Take sips of water and swish ("chew") it around in your mouth to activate hydrochloric acid for better digestion.
- Drink 8 ounces of quality water *before* each meal to assist in weight loss.
- Sip water throughout the whole day.
- Add fresh, sliced citrus or cucumbers to your water.
- Avoid drinking water from plastic bottles unless they are PBA free.
- Invest in a glass water bottle or water jug for daily water intake.

Step 9
Exercise – Move Like your Ancestors

In ancient times there was no mass transit, fancy smart phones or computers. Therefore, for purposes of communication, our ancient relatives naturally moved more than we do. People walked or climbed hills to have their needs met. Laundry was not sent out to the cleaners but was actually hand-washed and hung out to dry in the warm sun. Foods were harvested by hand through physical labor. Therefore, people performed more physical exercise and naturally moved their bodies.

1. Movement or exercise is very important to keep our bodies functioning properly. Moving our bodies means better circulation, blood flow, more oxygen intake and generally better well-being.
2. If you cannot join your local gym, I suggest you get outside in nature and walk, jog lightly (depending on your level of health and joint stability), go for a bike ride or swim.
3. If you belong to a gym, commit to a structured form of exercise three times per week. We should all incorporate some form of movement/exercise on a daily basis for at least thirty minutes.

Tips For Movement - Exercise

- Wake up earlier to make time for exercise.
- Stretch for 5-20 minutes before any workout.
- Join a health club or hire a certified fitness trainer.
- Take the stairs instead of an elevator.
- Park your car further away than normal to increase walking distance.
- Exercise with a buddy.
- Invest in an exercise video to do in the privacy of your own home.
- Walk or bike around your favorite area or neighborhood.
- Schedule and prioritize exercise for 30 minutes in your day.
- Choose activities you enjoy.
- Go for a gentle or moderate hike.
- Notice and accept your body's limitations and imbalances.
- See exercise as a fun and challenging opportunity. Think of exercise as "adult play time."
- Remind yourself of the importance of exercising and moving the body on a daily basis.

Step 10
Breathe In Life Force Energy

Breath is life. When you were born and came into this world, the first thing you did was breathe. If you don't breathe, you die – it is that simple.

1. The fact is: most people do not breathe properly. As part of a healthy lifestyle we need to be conscious of our breathing patterns and incorporate that consciousness into our daily lives.

2. Many people have an inverted breathing pattern; they breathe through the lungs instead of breathing from the belly and the diaphragm.

3. Improper breathing affects the body negatively, as it can restrict energy to the body and oxygen flow to the brain, organs and muscles.

4. Proper breathing creates more harmony in the body, mind and spirit, and general feelings of wellness, which help de-stress the body.

5. Correct breathing also creates more life force energy, leading to a more vibrant life.

Tips For Better Breathing

- Find a breathing buddy and schedule a breathing session together out in nature.
- Be conscious of your breath and practice breathing with awareness.
- Perform breath work after all meals to improve digestion.
- Lie down in a comfy spot and practice conscious breathing while placing your hands on your belly, being aware of your breath.
- Breathe through your nose with your mouth closed.
- Practice placing your tongue on the roof of your mouth, behind your two front teeth while breathing. This assists in opening up your diaphragm for better breathing capacity.
- Slow your breath down to induce relaxation.
- Pace yourself: inhale for 6 seconds and exhale for 6 seconds.
- Consider joining a chi gong or tai chi class to improve your breath intake.
- Breathe 2/3 oxygen into your belly, with the last 1/3 up through your diaphragm, and then your lungs.
- Allow 10 minutes minimum per day to practice breath work.

Step 11
Stretch Like The Animals

We should stretch EVERY DAY.

1. Animals innately stretch after a nap as a means to create more energy and wake up their bodies.

2. Stretching improves circulation and also awakens the body's energy systems and organs.

3. Some benefits of stretching include: greater flexibility, increased energy, expanded range of motion of the joints, less tension in the mind and body, plus blood flows with more ease to tight body parts.

4. Although, some experts advise to stretch in the evening, I prefer to perform my stretching routine upon awakening as I feel the energy flowing throughout my body awaking tight, sleepy muscles. I find stretching better than a cup of coffee.

Tips For Stretching

- Pick a comfy, uncluttered spot on the floor.
- Be aware of your breathing while stretching.
- Join a stretch class for guidance.
- Rent a stretching video.
- Stretch with the kids or a companion.
- Spend at least 20-minutes a day and/or evening stretching.
- Stretch to your favorite mellow music or an audio book.
- Focus on the muscles you are stretching.
- Wear comfy clothes.
- Stretch to the feeling of discomfort, NOT pain.
- Hold each posture for approximately 6 breaths or 30 seconds before releasing the stretch.
- Breathe in through the nose and out through the nose.
- Place your tongue on the roof of your mouth behind your teeth to assist in bringing more oxygen to the stretched muscles.
- Schedule your stretch sessions.

Step 12
Strengthen and Tone Your Temple

As we age, we naturally lose functional muscle-tone. Therefore, it is extremely important to incorporate an exercise routine well into your golden years. Our bodies were designed to live long, prosperous lives as long as we care for them properly.

1. You were not meant to succumb to wheelchairs and walkers. In indigenous cultures, wheelchairs and walkers do not exist. I trust that is due to the movement the elders are getting on a daily basis; walking, hiking, doing outdoor chores and moving.

2. I am not suggesting you move to the Andes or Himalayas, but I am suggesting you begin – at any age – to condition your body through strength and conditioning exercises.

3. A strong, vibrant physique has better posture, is more functional, creates higher confidence levels and a better general sense of well-being.

Tips For Strengthening Your Body

- Sign up for a group strength and conditioning class at your local gym.
- Rent or purchase a basic exercise video and perform the routine at home.
- Schedule exercise for 3 days per week.
- Hire a certified personal trainer or coach for guidance.
- Consider doing compound exercises (a compound exercise is working more than one muscle group at the same time while performing one exercise).
- Be very present to the muscles you are working during exercise/movement.
- Exercise ALL muscles for a balanced exercise routine.
- Alternate aerobic and weighted exercise and don't forget stretches.
- Buy some light or moderately heavy weights to work your prime muscles (legs, arms, thighs, chest, stomach and back).
- Purchase various size rocks or small boulders from your local quarry or home improvement/tile store and move rocks around your back yard or make rock stacks.
- Always be aware of your posture while exercising.

Step 13
Forgiveness – Letting Go Of Anger

There may be one, two or several people in your life whom you feel you may need to forgive. It is my experience that lack of forgiveness creates lack of peace of mind. In my opinion, lack of peace of mind creates dis-ease and illness.

1. Why would one want to hold a grudge and carry negative emotions throughout their lifetime? After all, it is only ourselves we are harming – emotionally, physically and mentally.
2. Research shows forgiveness can: create a deeper spirituality; relieve stress and depression; ease physical pain; improve sleep and lower blood pressure.
3. Lack of forgiveness and non-acceptance drains the positive life force energy from the body. Remember that holding onto anger is not healthy and creates stress and dis-ease in the body.
4. In today's harried and chaotic world, we need all the positive life force we can muster to sustain vibrant health and wellness.

Tips For Forgiveness & Releasing Anger

- Be aware of your response or reaction.
- Go outside and breathe before you respond or react.
- Take a walk to diffuse anger.
- Pray to God, your higher power or Great Spirit and ask your higher self for the strength to forgive.
- Pray for the person whom you feel wronged you and needs forgiveness.
- Send loving thoughts to the person you feel needs forgiveness.
- Write a letter asking for forgiveness, read it, feel it, then burn it or throw it in the trash. Let it go!
- Treat and forgive others as you would want them to treat and forgive you.
- Since you can't change it, let go of the past as it no longer serves you.
- Remind yourself that NO ONE is perfect, including the person whom you choose not to forgive.
- Release some anger through an exercise session.

Step 14

Purpose - Why Do You Exist?

Did you ever wonder why you were born? Is there a part of you that wonders what your purpose and dream is? It is my belief, if we have no purpose on this earth, we are merely existing.

1. Once we discover our purpose and begin to dream of its inherent possibilities, we have a reason to live and not merely exist. We have a purposeful reason to get out of bed in the morning – a reason to live in love and joy.

2. If finances were not an issue and you had all the money to meet your needs, what would you choose to do? How would you choose to spend your time? What is your heart's desire?

3. Consider what your legacy will be and work toward that legacy. How would you like to be remembered at your funeral? What would you want your legacy to be... what would you like to leave to the world?

4. I suggest you consider your deepest desire, set a powerful intention in your mind and heart to fulfill your destiny - and live your purpose and dream.

5. Remember, energy follows intent.

Tips To Discovering Your Purpose And Dream

- Practice loving yourself unconditionally.
- Think about and discover what you've always loved and wanted to do.
- Take baby steps that head in the direction of living your purpose and dream.
- Hire a professional life coach to assist you in discovering your dream.
- Envision what you love – see it in your mind's eye and feel it in your heart.
- Find a support group.
- Find a good book on discovering your life's purpose; buy it, read it and work toward creating your dream.
- Start a daily journal and log daily activities and/or hobbies which bring you closer to your dream and purpose.
- Create a vision board to reflect your desires and dreams.
- Join a Mastermind group (a group to help you handle challenges).
- Watch an inspirational movie.
- Learn to believe in yourself.
- Surround yourself with like-minded individuals who have a similar purpose and dream.

Step 15
Joy – Live Life to Its Fullest

The meaning of joy: "the emotion of great delight or happiness caused by something exceptionally good or satisfying; keen pleasure; elation."

1. What does joy mean to you? I realize we all have different definitions of joy due to our own unique experiences.
2. What would it mean for you to live a joyful life? I suggest it would mean a person who lived a satisfying and fulfilling life had no regrets.
3. Perhaps you are currently experiencing true joy. What brings you joy?
4. Would you consider digging deep to ponder this question?
5. Ok, now that you figured out what truly brings you joy, go after that joy and live your life to the fullest!

Tips For Living A More Joyful Life

- Practice being at peace with yourself.
- Learn to open your heart to everyone, as we are all ONE.
- Smile often – offer a smile to a stranger.
- Dance like no one is watching.
- Be honest with everyone, starting with YOU.
- Practice being polite to all.
- Don't spend money on things you can't afford.
- Spend time with joyful, happy people.
- Avoid depressed, negative, energy-sapping individuals.
- Let yourself cry when you feel sad.
- Reconnect with nature.
- Expand your mind with knowledge.
- Practice being present with all you do.
- Cuddle with a loved one, precious friend, favorite pet, family member or child.
- Stop and literally "smell the roses".
- Laugh more.
- Learn to love and accept yourself as perfectly imperfect.
- Love and accept all.

I trust you will find these tips beneficial for your health, wellness and fitness journey. Thank you for taking the first step or steps towards a new you!

You've finished. Before you go...

<u>Tweet/share that you finished this book.</u>

Please star rate this book.

Reviews are solid gold to writers. Please take a few minutes to give us some itty bitty feedback on this book.

ABOUT THE AUTHOR

Patricia Garza Pinto is a certified CHEK Holistic Lifestyle Coach and CHEK Corrective Exercise Specialist. Patricia is certified by world renown Holistic Health Practitioner, Paul Chek, in Corrective Holistic Exercise Kinesiology.

Patricia is also a Reiki Practitioner and Shamanic Energy Medicine Healer. In addition, Patricia carries national fitness certifications from the American College of Sports Medicine (ACSM) and the American Council on Exercise (ACE).

Patricia has 42 years of fitness and exercise experience and approaches wellness from many perspectives, integrating them into a unified whole...mind, body and spirit.

For more information about her programs, visit:
www.divinemountainretreat.com

Patricia Garza Pinto, President & Founder
Divine Mountain Retreat
949-422-1168
www.divinemountainretreat.com
patriciawholistic@gmail.com

If you enjoyed this Itty Bitty® book you might also like…

- **Your Amazing Itty Bitty® Aging Well Book** – Michele McHenry

- **Your Amazing Itty Bitty® Self-Care Book** – Denise Schickel

- **Your Amazing Itty Bitty® Health and Wellness Experts Compilation Book** – Various Authors

Or any of the many Amazing Itty Bitty® books available on line at www.ittybittypublishing.com